Sunday Night Knife & Gun Club

by L.S. Collison

Episode #3

Nurse Kit Carson's Adventures

America's New Wild West

Cover design by M.G. Manelis

ISBN: 978-1-7322290-2-0 (paperback)
ISBN: 978-1-7322290-1-3 (electronic edition)
Fiction House, Ltd.
Steamboat Springs, Colorado

With special thanks to Gloria
and the gang
who taught me to ride & rope

Sunday Night

Kit Carson

The winter had been a long one and it was not yet spring. I was driving to work, late

again, mind busy, overflowing with to-do lists, should-have-done lists, the

occasional misplaced memory blowing through like a random tumbleweed. Last

week's lynching, the way the dead man's boots twitched, a dog dreaming. Tonto's

forearms, his concentration when he drew his bow (a warm tingling down south,

picturing his muscles tensed, the arrow poised). Those men we left for dead down

in the hospital morgue. Random images. Floaters. Blink, they're gone and a new day's

shit pile to deal with.

My pickup, a Dodge Power Wagon, galloping along with never a word of

complaint. Oil change and new tires all the way around – that put a dent in my

charge card but I felt indestructible in that badass machine. Love my sexy set of wheels, she's fully restored (except for a broken window and glove box latch) and only five more years of payments! Lately, a family had taken up residence in the back, hanging a blue plastic tarp over the bed, tent-like, to keep out the sleet and snow. Beneath the tarp a string of lights lent a bit of cheer to the situation. I'd never actually seen any of them, they were invisible to me, but I couldn't help notice little scraps of their existence. A glove dropped in the snow. An empty water bottle under the wheel. Sometimes when I got into the cab I smelled green chili and pork simmering in the back. But I kept my blinders on. Hell, I had enough to worry about looking after my own. Those people were no concern of mine.

Traffic in town was heavy that Sunday night, a regular stampede. Used to be Sundays were slow but lately there'd been a rush of interlopers to the city of High Plains and the whole Front Range. They came for the silver, they came for the gold, they came for the oil and gas, they come for the dope. It's boom or bust baby, and High Plains was booming. Me, I'm practically a native, I've got the bumper sticker to prove it.

I stepped on the gas and was making up for lost time when I saw a lasso of blue and red lights in the rearview. Shit damn hellsafire, I don't need this.

Braking and signaling (and hoping my lights weren't burned out), I pulled off the highway onto the shoulder. What will I say? Cops and nurses, we supposedly have an affinity or something. I'll tell him I'm late for my shift and give him the look, you know the look. Maybe I'll get lucky and he'll let me off. Unless... What if it's one of Bully Ratzer's deputies? What if he knows the dancer Balmy Wether is under *my* protection, that she's living under my roof, babysitting my kids, taking online courses to get her high school diploma? What if he knows she's ready to rat out the sheriff of High Plains?

A flashlight in my face, a tap on the window. "Roll 'em down, cowgirl."

My stomach, in knots. "It won't roll down," I said, speaking loudly, so he could hear me through the glass. "It's broken. The window's broken."

"Keep your hands where I can see 'em."

I gripped the steering wheel to keep my hands from shaking.

"Now open the door. Easy does it, nice and slow. Keep your right hand on the wheel."

I did as he bid.

"Atta girl."

The hombre was tall. Over six feet, I reckoned. I couldn't even see his face way up there.

"Now, let me see your papers. Driver's license, registration, proof of insurance. No sudden moves, cowgirl. "

The click of a safety being released triggered my heart rate to 130 sinus tach, with a couple of PVCs thrown in. I could accurately gauge its rate and rhythm because heartbeats are my business. Critical care and emergency nursing, my expertise. Swallowing hard, I reached over to open the glove box and the damn door fell off in my hand. Of course it did; I had forgotten about the broken latch. Out poured an avalanche of shit – old gasoline receipts, unopened pack of tampons and an empty pack of Marlboros, CPR pocket mask, a box of nine millimeter bullets and a wad of paper napkins from Waco Taco. Somewhere amid the detritus of my road life I found what I was looking for. Handed over my paperwork and awaited my fate.

He shone the flashlight on my card. "Your insurance is expired."

"Well, actually it's not. I just keep forgetting to replace the card."

"Ma'am, this card is ten years old."

"It is? But really I do have car insurance, officer."

"Yeah? Well, what about health insurance. You got that?"

"Can't afford it. I'm a per diem nurse. No bennies. Gig economy, ya know?"

"It looks like I'm going to have to write you up, cowgirl. Wait here 'til I run this." The lawman went back to his ride. Shit, I am fucked. They're probably done with report by now; I'm liable to get the boot for being late again.

Meanwhile, cars flew by me on the highway. I could just imagine the drivers looking over and seeing me snared by the blue and red lasso, thinking "serves her right" and "better her than me." Altruism is dead.

The cop wasn't gone long, and when he came back he handed me an envelope. "Be careful now, Nurse Carson," he said. "Be real careful. You're being watched."

My stomach tightened, and the skin on the back of my neck tingled. "Thank you, Officer," I said. "I'll be on the lookout." For what, I wondered?

He turned to go then paused, looking over his shoulder. "I see you're carrying undocumented workers."

"I am?" I feigned surprise. "But I've never actually *seen* anyone back there."

The officer touched the brim of his hat. "Well, ma'am, I'll be on my way. Take care now."

He walked off into the moonlight, his boots crunching on the gravel. Got in his ride and waited for me to drive off.

It wasn't until I got to work, parked in the lot, that I dared open the envelope. Right there in the parking garage, I read it under the sickly yellow lights.

You are hereby requested to appear at the Watering Hole Saloon, Sunday night at

9:00 pm.

Come alone and come armed.

~ High Plains Vigilantes for American Justice

My stomach did a flip- flop, my fingertips tingled. Carefully I put the slip of paper back in the envelope and stuffed it inside my Kevlar vest. There must be some mistake. Not to mention, the Watering Hole was such a dive. Only the drovers and the dregs drank there.

*

Halliday

Dr. Ruth Halliday slipped into the nurses' lounge for a cuppa joe before starting her shift. The little room, the so-called "lounge," (really more of a burrow or a den) was a mélange of ethnic food odors, microwave popcorn, coffee, and something else – what was it? – wet socks? The nurses were a messy lot, but they had coffee. Real brew, an old- fashioned communal coffee pot, which was more than she could say for the doctors' lounge, which actually *was* a lounge, a well-appointed one, but way over in the south wing. Not that anyone thought ER doctors needed a lounge. In the eyes of the head honchos, Emergency physicians were glorified veterinarians. Whatever, she didn't care. She was just putting in her time here. At least in the nurses' den she had her own coffee cup. The nurses had bought it for her last Christmas and filled it with chocolate hearts and candy kisses. They even had it personalized with her name:

Doc Halliday

Badass-est ER Doc in the West

The mug was stained with a little chip out of the handle. Damaged, like the nurses. She loved them. They were almost like family. No, they were family.

Pulling her slouch hat low over one eye, Ruth adjusted her thigh holsters beneath the canvas duster she had taken to wearing and looped the stethoscope around her neck with a practiced flip of her hand. Pushed the swinging door open and went out to face the night.

A glance at the white board in the nurses' station was a preview of the night to come.

Rm. 1 Johnson FLU SX OTD

Rm. 2 Chang Ψ consult

Rm. 3 Miller FUO ADMT RM #602

Rm. 4 Barnes LOLNAD FOS?

Rm. 5 Garcia SOB

Rm. 6 Gonzales R/O FX R radius OTD

Rm. 7 Walsh ETOH BA? (316 Bess 288 Shorty 250 Larry)

The ER hands wrote and spoke a language of initials and acronyms. It was a shorthand and a code as well as a psychological buffer. Must maintain a distance even while we are invading their bodies and minds with fingers, tubes, catheters, sharp instruments, blunt words.

"Howdy, Doc Ruth." Stretch, the EMT, a cocky little cowhand but a good kid; a team player. "Better place your bet on Walsh's BA before the labs come back, ma'am."

The ER staff runs pools, bets on lab results, especially blood alcohol levels; those were the favored game. Were they frequent fliers? If so, there's a baseline BA on them in the medical records and the player places his bet comparing the patient's current LOC with past levels of consciousness. The nurses run this casino, but the docs are inveterate gamblers, everyone knows. Ruth was always game to play along.

OTD on only two rooms. *Out the Door.* Discharged. Treat 'em and street 'em, that's our goal. LOLNAD always a favorite, those sweet little old ladies in no apparent distress. A memory of baking cookies with Gramma flashes through her consciousness except there were no smells of baking cookies to accompany the visual. Instead another scent, a warm chocolate mess but definitely not chocolate chips, she'd wager.

TVs blaring, every monitor in the department tuned to the corporate Wellmart channel, all they could get. Be glad when this election's over, sick of the political stink. Bully Ratzer promising to make the West wild again, guaranteeing freedom and gun rights for all. His ads were all over the media, his face on posters and handbills all over town. Running against the righteously shrill-voiced Marjorie Bledsoe. Maybe she did sell arms to the Arapahos and, yeah, the last Comanche attack happened on her watch, but Ratzer's a lying, thieving, extorting, uneducated bounder. Bad enough he's sheriff – Can't believe he's running for governor. But no way he'll win, not after we expose him. In this country a man's character counts for something.

*

Room 4. Pull on gloves, insert finger into anus, mind far away. Mind divided, split screen. One side, an old white woman's hind end; on the other, Ruth's happy place, a Las Vegas casino, where the piano man plays a lively tune and the smell of whiskey and fine cigars fill the air. In her hand, a royal flush.

The hostess with perky boobs brings her drink, her musky perfume has a lingering finish…

On the gurney the patient twisted and bucked like a steer, crying rape. Whoa Nelly, hold still there, we're trying to help you. The nurse struggled to hold the old woman down. Carson, that's her name. Kit Carson. She's the one mixed up in the whole Wether sisters affair.

Ruth extracted her finger, wiped it on the disposable pad and peeled the gloves off, one encased neatly inside the other. She then dropped the wad of latex into the biohazard trash.

"Disempact her, nurse Carson. Clean 'er out real good. Test for occult blood, just for the record, and send her back to the home."

What people don't realize is a fecal impaction can kill you. Slowly. Insidiously. But as surely as a bullet in the brain, shit stuck in the colon can kill. Another life saved. Yippi ty yi yay, get along little doggie, it's your misfortune and none of my own.

*

Kit

"You're late, Carson," the charge nurse had accused. "Report was finished ten minutes ago."

"Sorry," I said. "I got pulled over by the Law."

"Sorry don't cut it; it'll be noted on your record. But here's your chance for redemption. Tonight, every shit patient is yours; starting with room 4." She flashed me a jaded smirk. "Oh, and you'll want the heavy duty gloves. Extra long."

That's how I got stuck with the dis-impaction. Halliday, of course, didn't stick around for all of that. Digging out is a nurse's job. A new pack of blue plastic pads, a tube of lubricant, a bag of warm water hanging from the IV pole, I was ready to go.

"Unhand me, bitch!" Little Old Lady cried out, imperious as a queen.

"Whoa there, Nellie! Hold still, this won't take long." One hand on her bony hip, I steeled myself for the task.

"Alexa, play something soothing."

Oh, give me land, lots of land under starry skies above, Gene Autry crooned.

"Alexa, turn up the volume."

Fifteen minutes later, the dirty deed done, I opened a vial of peppermint oil to freshen the air. The descending colon was now glistening pink and empty, and the woman to whom the organ belonged was sleeping. Come morning, this would all be an unpleasant dream for both of us.

I made my exit, carrying a blue bundle of steaming shit in my hands. The hallway was lined with spectators – families of other patients in adjoining rooms – who had undoubtedly heard everything going on behind the curtain. They watched me in horror as I made my way toward the hopper, dumped the load and flushed twice.

Back in the patient's room, Ruth was doing a final check.

"You were invited," she said to me. It was a statement. Definitely not a question.

"I was what?"

She didn't respond but glanced pointedly toward the camera mounted above the door. You couldn't be too careful, there were eyes and ears everywhere.

"Alexa, get me Mr. Smith's medical records. And play *I'm an Old Cowhand.*"

When the music started, she spoke in a low, matter-of-fact voice, like she was asking me to open a packet of KY jelly. "You were invited to the watering hole Sunday night. We could use a few good nurses." She pulled a prescription pad out of her pocket, scribbled something, tore it off and gave it to me. *Meet us at the blackjack table at nine, ready to roll*

"It's a shooting club," she said with a look freighted with hidden meaning. "We get together for cards and drinks."

Ruth Halliday, that old buffalo soldier, was a vigilante?

I figured maybe I should go. I wasn't very good at shooting, my marksmanship

sucked, but I could stick a vein, any vein, on the first try. Blindfolded, one hand

behind my back. If there was a medal for IV sticks, I'd a won it. Good at triage too.

Maybe those skills would come in handy. Hopefully they weren't looking for a

secretary. I had never been a joiner, my social life was null and void, and I hadn't a

clue how to play blackjack. But I had been asked – tapped – by a secret society. It

was flattering, it was an honor. I only hoped the dues wouldn't be too high.

*

Wyatt

He hit PAUSE, freezing the game. His eyes hurt. He was hungry, or bored. Maybe

both. Calamity, asleep on the couch next to Balmy, season 36 of *The Gamblers* on

the screen. So boring it must have knocked them out. He was lonely but didn't want

to wake them, especially not his sister; she would be all needy and want him to

make popcorn. Wait – popcorn – good idea. They looked like unborn babies, all fetal

together, eyelids fluttering, minds blank. Unidentical twins. Fraternal twins. No,

sisternal twins. Except Balmy's not my sister. I don't know how long she's gonna

stay with us. I like her – she's hot – even if her face is all fucked up from the

beatings.

But something's not right. The hair on the back of his neck prickled. Gun up, make the rounds. Check windows. Check doors and locks. Still, the feeling, the sharp taste in his mouth. I'm the man of the house. Protector.

What's that? Sounds like something's up in the crawl space. Squirrels? A raccoon? Maybe an intruder. The piece, solid in his hand. Safety off, the bitch was ready. Do a visual on every room, check all five. Maybe a minute passed. Maybe more. All quiet.

Fuck! Somebody was knocking at the door! No, not a knock, more like a soft tap-tap-tap. He stood on his toes to look out the peephole but couldn't see anything. Another tap-tap-tap. Just do it, go on. Safety off, he was ready for anything. Ready to squeeze the trigger and blow the sumbitch away.

There at his feet, a puppy. No shit, a real live puppy all shivering and pathetic. As Wyatt bent to scoop it up, he saw the boy standing in the shadows of the porch. His own height. No hat. No fucking hat. Shivering like the puppy. With the door open the wind blew in, swirling through the house. But the boy just stood there. Wyatt thought he looked familiar.

"This your dog?"

"I thought you might want it."

The kid sounded alright. Sounded normal. Wyatt judged him not a threat. The puppy squirmed and he felt a sudden wet warmth against his stomach.

"Come on in," he said, his hands full with puppy and gun. "Take your shoes off; my mom'll have a fit."

The boy removed his off-brand sneakers and lined them up next to the others in the boot tray beside the door. Wyatt put his finger to his lips. Now the gun felt awkward and stupid, but he didn't want to lay it down, not just yet. He motioned for the boy to follow him to his bedroom where he shut the door behind them so they could talk.

"Are you one of the ones who live in the back of our truck?"

The kid nodded.

"What's your name?"

"Mike. What's yours?"

"Wyatt. What are you doing here?"

"Relocating. My dad and my uncle are looking for work."

"What kind of work?"

"Wiring houses 'n stuff. They're electricians."

"You speak good English."

The boy named Mike looked at him, like, duh. "Born in the U.S.A. Same as you."

Wyatt was aware of the puppy, chewing his fingers with tiny, sharp teeth. He could smell his sour puppy breath and his puppy pee on his shirt. "What should we name him?"

Mike shrugged. "What about Cesar?"

"Yeah, that's cool. I think Cesar's hungry. What about you?"

Mike smiled.

"Me too. Let's make some popcorn."

*

Kit

Hospitals and bars each have their own particular stink. Frankly, I preferred the lived-in smell of a local watering hole. That smoky, whiskey, wet leather and beer-soaked floorboards funk was a welcome change from the hospital's olfactory delights. I'd never spent much time in the company of drinkers, but I'd always wanted to be part of the easy camaraderie, the low society of alcoholics, whores, gamblers, cocaine dealers and piano players who call a bar home.

I sat at the blackjack table, next to Doc; I was in deep over my head after only an hour. The barmaid had just brought another round when my phone vibrated. A text from Wyatt, I read it discreetly under the table.

Mom, can I have a dog?

No. Go to sleep.

I found one by the front door. He was cold.

No dogs, Wyatt.

Mom?

What?

The boy's name is Mike.

What boy?

You know. The boy who lives in the back of the truck.

Don't encourage them! Be safe, keep doors locked, guns loaded! Good Night!

I added a bunch of hearts and zzzzz's to sign off.

Mentally back in the game, but now I had lost my focus and any luck I might have had. I couldn't help feeling out of my element. I didn't even know these people. Well, except for Doc Halliday and Officer True who had pulled me over last week. High rollers, hired guns, and card sharps by the looks of it. I fingered my little stack of chips and tried to concentrate.

The dealer shuffled the cards and began a new session. Wait, what? Graffiti on the cards. Words and cryptic phrases. My assignment was turning up bit by bit on the faces of the cards. A seven of spades with "Balmy" scrawled in pencil. A queen of diamonds said "Stormy Wether in Cheyenne." So this is how it's played! My breath came in gulps but I put on my best poker face. Played a card, was dealt

another. The deuce of clubs. Across its face in black ink. *Fold 'em sucker!*

I looked at Doc and she nodded. I stood up, leaving my chips, my cards on the

table. "I got you covered," Halliday said. And so I walked out into the cold night,

trying to piece it all together, what I was expected to do.

The doctor caught up with me in the parking lot.

"Tonto's got Stormy, he's expecting you at the Hitching Post on Lincoln Avenue.

His people have agreed to give the sisters refuge until after the story breaks and

Ratzer's taken down. But don't expect it to go smoothly. We have reason to believe

the plan's been hacked."

I reached for my keys, a tingle of fear and excitement racing through my arms

and legs.

"Wait a minute," Doc said. "I've got some medical supplies. Never know what

you're going to run into out there."

Halliday went to her ride and brought back a medical kit, must've weighed

twenty pounds. I took a look inside: antibiotics, catheters and ET tubes, enema

kits, IV supplies, scalpels, pick-ups, sutures, splints. All the essential drugs, even a

flask of whiskey and a bite stick. Hell, with these supplies I could dig out a bullet,

deliver a breech calf, or transplant a kidney. I was set.

"Anything else I need to know?"

"There'll be a reporter from the Washington Post with the Indians, to interview the sisters. When this story hits the papers, Bully Ratzer's going down."

From the back of my truck I could hear music. Very faint, but yes, it was definitely mariachi. I fired up the ignition, wondering if Halliday heard it.

"Keep your cell phone handy. Plans could change at any minute." The doctor started to walk back to the bar then paused, looking over her shoulder.

"*Vaya con Dios*, Carson."

*

Tonto

He had been following the white owl for miles, westward across the plain. Whether the raptor was real in feather and flesh or existed only in his mind's eye, he couldn't say. Didn't matter, it was one and the same. Mile after mile after mile, astride the steel and chrome Indian Chief Dark Horse rumbling through the night, Tim Rhodes, a.k.a. Tonto, rode like the wind along the ancient pathway of his people. I-80. A pathway now paved with asphalt and divided by white slashes, like war paint.

He rode in a trance-like state, unmindful of the biting wind on his cheek, dreaming in the old language, a language he had never been taught yet somehow understood. He was getting aroused, the vibration of his motorcycle between his legs, the woman's arms around him, her warm breasts pressing into his back, her bruised face resting against his shoulder. Couldn't help that. He may be Arapaho, he may be a nurse, but he was a man first and foremost. Not so young anymore, his hair gone to gray, but he was still virile. Was Stormy sleeping, he wondered? He hoped so. Tonto felt gentle and powerful at the same time. He would fight, he would kill if he had to, though it violated his oath. He was, after all, a nurse. A rogue nurse but still a nurse who lived by the sacred creed. *Do no harm, take no shit.*

Ahead, the white owl circled impatiently, waiting for him to catch up.

The road stretched ahead, rising slightly with each mile. No moon tonight, only starlight, the voices of a million lives, past lives, lives yet to come. Certainly he had entertained fantasies of Stormy, what man hadn't? But now that she was under his protection it was the other female, the one back in High Plains whom he was thinking of. The nurse who called herself Kit Carson, he imagined she had been sent by the spirit Splinter-foot, the huntress born of the hunter's swollen leg. Tonto had been studying Arapaho mythology, having been deprived of it growing up. Splinter-foot lived with her six sisters in a star cluster high overhead, what the dominant culture called the Pleiades or Seven Sisters. Tonto lived close to the

stars.

They were at war with Nihancan, the crazy one, the spider trickster, that old

enemy of the White Sage People. Nihancan was the white man with the gun. Tonto

was only now coming into the fullness of understanding, awareness of his being, his

true *being*. White Owl and Splinter-Foot were his spirit guides. His mission

unfolded before him. To deliver the dancing woman and her sister to the safety

and protection of his people, waiting for him in Cheyenne.

Ahead, the owl flew on like an arrow, time's arrow, and beneath him his ride

rumbled on.

*

Kit

Hauling ass on the highway, heading north. Searching for a radio station, but it's all

shit these days. The clutter on the edge of town, never ending. Once endless plains

and open range, now condos and swimming pools, outlet malls and superstores,

ranchettes and golf courses. They keep coming, all looking for something, for blue

sky and purple sage. Everybody wants to be a cowboy, baby. Everybody wants to

get high and shoot a gun.

One eye on the rearview, I've got a feeling I'm being followed. Ratzer's men are everywhere, or so I imagined. It's a damn shame we can't trust our elected public servants.

"Mommy, I'm hungry."

"Hang on, sweetheart. Balmy, would you kindly get her a pop tart? They're in my saddle bag."

I could feel the teenager's eye roll in the dark. She exhaled a sigh of forbearance and reached down on the floor by her feet to oblige me.

"No need to be rude, Balmy. Where are your manners?"

"Yes, *ma'am.*"

"No need to be sarcastic either. A little gratitude would be appreciated, thank you." I liked her. She reminded me of me, a few years back. All hair and attitude with tits to match.

It was Balmy who got Stormy to the hospital after the sheriff's goons tried to convince Stormy to keep silent. It was really Balmy who saved Stormy's life. After her operation, the vigilantes had her airlifted to an undisclosed private facility in Kansas to recover. There, she had been given a new identity. But none of us would rest until Bully and his men were behind bars.

From the back seat I could hear the music leaking from Wyatt's earbuds.

"Turn that down, cowboy, you're going to blow out your eardrums."

Amazingly, he complied. Then I heard another sound, a whimpering whine that could only be one thing.

"Is there a dog in my back seat?"

No answer, just another pathetic sound like a small, helpless animal pleading for its life.

"I told you no dogs."

"He needs a home, Mommy," says Calamity. "He lost his family."

Don't look, I tell myself. But I do. One quick glance in the rearview is enough. Oh, that little fucker. So small, so helpless, so stinkin' cute.

"Goddammit, kids. Last thing in the world I need is a puppy chewing my boots. Last thing I need is to step in a puddle in my stocking feet. Last thing I need is another creature depending on me for their very existence." My turn to heave a sigh, which no one comprehended or even heard.

The smell of acetone filled the cab. Next to me, Balmy was painting her nails, her hand splayed out on her denim-clad thigh. Her long dancer's legs folded at impossible angles, her stocking feet on the seat next to her ass. She resembled the letter M. Her hair cascaded over her shoulders. Balmy's been a sex slave who knows how long? I wondered what her real name was but I didn't ask. All of us hide behind our avatars.

"Hey, Balms," said Wyatt from the back seat. "Pass me the pop tarts, bee-atch."

They maligned each other lovingly, like brother and sister.

"Wait a sec, butthead, my nails are wet." She blew on her fingertips like she was extinguishing sixteen birthday candles on a cake. Tossed the box of tarts into the back seat. In the rearview, I saw Wyatt slide open the window and pass the box through to the waiting hand on the other side. So he was feeding them too.

Balmy, finished with her manicure, made a pillow of my saddlebag and fell asleep against the window. It amazed me how quickly she could tune out the world. The kids in the back, the puppy, all quiet. Not a peep. I was in charge; they all trusted me to keep them safe while they slept. Jesusfuckingchrist, the responsibility was overwhelming sometimes. But the hum of tires against the asphalt was liberating. Behind us, the city lights fell away and the darkness swallowed us. Now I could see a scattering of stars through the windshield. One of them was the North Star but which one? The night sky was a revolving map, but I didn't know how to read it. If it wasn't for my phone I'd be lost. Tonto would know. Tonto, on his way to meet us, our paths to intersect. Maybe after the Wether sisters were safely reunited he and I would unite. The thought warmed me as I imagined the details. Mile after mile the highway unfurled.

*

Out of nowhere, headlights were creeping up my ass. I got an odd feeling, I don't know, like I get when a patient who looks stable is fixin' to go south. Call it intuition, call it luck, call it experience. I gave the beast a kick in the gas flanks and sped up to ninety to see if I could lose whoever was tailing me, but they kept up. Then I slowed back down, thinking, what if it's the Law and they're after me for speeding? But there was no lasso of lights, no siren. The hair on my arms stood up. Suddenly I'm scared shitless, I need some help here! Buck up, Carson. Keep your hands on the wheel and your foot on the gas.

*

Calamity

Was it too late to be someone else? If she went to sleep, might she dream up a new life? Next life she would have a dad like the one in the dollhouse. That dad had gone missing too, it was her fault. *Calamity, keep your toys picked up!* Sad. Suck on the blanket's soft corner. *Close your eyes and go to sleep, Calamity.* Fake sleep. Play dead to survive, that's what they taught in school. Fire drills and shooter drills. Stranger danger, Sharing is caring. When you wish upon a star. ABCDEFG.

Wyatt's friend, his family, those Electricans that live in the back of the truck, they'll help us, we'll help them. Just like a real family, a family with a dad or maybe even two.

*

Balmy

She had somehow lost her memories, maybe left them in a dream. Now she was in a dream, knew she was dreaming. Looking for something or someone. Her sister. Not Stormy but her real sister, possibly her identical twin. She wanted to call out to her, but she couldn't remember her name. She couldn't remember her own name. A door, she opened it, a swinging barroom door, and inside, a mechanical girl on all fours, twisting and bucking for all she was worth. Sign said *Drop a nickel in the Slot to make her Buck.* The next cowboy climbed on. She looked up and smiled, but her face was a cow's skull, bleached white bone, empty sockets for eyes.

"Balmy!"

Now she's grabbing the mechanical girl by the hair, pulling with all her might, struggling toward the surface of the dream. Wanting to breathe.

"Balmy, wake up!"

*

Kit

"Balmy, you awake?"

She mumbled something from behind the curtain of bleached hair.

"Balmy, wake up. Trouble behind and it ain't Casey Jones."

The teenager unfolded herself, now wide awake.

"Somebody's tailing us. I don't like the looks of it." Was it just some Wyoming

cowboy on meth? Or was it one of Ratzer's posse in pursuit?

The lights in my rearview flashed on high beam, nearly blinding me. I signaled,

moving over into the slow lane, to allow them to pass, but they followed, staying

right up my ass. I tromped my boot on the accelerator, and my Power Wagon leaped

like a charger, the speedometer pegged at 110. We charged along the highway,

straight as an arrow. I moved back into the fast lane, though there were no cars

ahead of me as far as I could see. Fort Collins was now behind us, we were entering

the territory's north forty. Gone were the strip malls, the condominium clones, the

big box stores. It was like driving into the past, into the real American West. Still,

the vehicle behind me kept pace.

"Now hold on in the back, kids, and get ready. I'm fixin' to flip a bitch."

Easing up on the gas, slowing down until I knew I could pull it off, I suddenly

veered across the median strip. Up onto two wheels, bouncing on the rough turf, I held my breath until I hit the southbound pavement, finishing my turn. From the back, yeehaws and *arribas* as we flew past the vehicle on our tail, a late model luxury SUV, black or possibly gray, hard to tell. In my rearview, I saw the brake lights as they slowed, probably preparing to make the same maneuver. Turned my headlights off, down-shifted to slow my speed so the brake lights wouldn't show, then drove onto the shoulder, past the guardrail and onto the frontage road, took it to the next overpass, crossed over and headed north again on the east access road, driving like hellfire, no lights. Quite a piece of fancy ridin' if I do say so myself.

"Mommy, I have to tinkle."

"Hold it, Calamity. I'm a little busy here."

"But I've been holding it a long time already."

"Mom, are we there yet?" Wyatt, coming to life again in the back seat.

"We can't outrun these guys forever, they've got a faster horse. Besides, we're low on gas. Balmy, pull up a map, would you? See what our options are. Find some place to lose these losers."

Next to me, Balmy studied the screen in the palm of her hand. In her lap I saw my revolver, locked and loaded. "There's a ghost town ahead to the right. Further right – I mean East – you can pick up 85."

Lights behind us on the frontage road, are you fucking kidding me? I dug my spurs into the floorboard, urging the old Wagon on.

"Or," said Balmy, "there's the sandstone fort ahead, just off the interstate. Maybe we can ambush 'em."

"Text Tonto, tell him to meet us there, pronto. Tell him what to expect. Wyatt, cover your sister. Keep your heads down. But just in case, you better gun up the guys in the back."

Wyatt took the Remington off the gun rack and handed it back through the sliding panel.

The bad guys fired first (they always do.) The sound of bullets ricocheting off the Wagon's flanks.

"Get down and stay down!" I slammed the pedal to the metal, the last bit of speed out of the beast, watching the gas gauge drop almost to E.

My phone pinged with an incoming text.

"Tonto," Balmy announced. "He's on his way."

*

A pop, a lurch, and suddenly it felt like we were driving through a river of sand. Tire blown, probably shot out. Like a bad dream, I fought for control. We were crippled, hobbled, no chance of outrunning them now. I needed a little time, but time had run out.

I smelled gasoline. What the hell? From the back of the truck I heard a loud crash, the breaking of glass. In my mirrors a flash of light followed by the force of an explosion, like a tailwind from hell, followed by an unholy boom.

"Hooray! It's the Electricans," Wyatt called out. I felt a burst of gratitude for the family in the back, the people I had chosen not to see. We were in this together, our lives were all at stake. Firebombs made with recycled bottles and gas from the red can, buying us a little time and sending out a signal of distress. Get the kids to safety, the only thought on my mind. Keep driving. Bumping along on three good tires and a rim, putting distance between us. Ahead, I could see the towering sandstone hoodoos, glowing red in the fire's light, offering their silent protection.

*

We stepped carefully over the bones and broken arrow shafts, shards of booze bottles crunching underfoot, looking for a place to hide. Wyatt and Mike found a snug little cavity in the rock, just above eye level. The kids climbed up, snuggling in like a little wolf pack, the puppy nestled between them. A silver-haired woman with a machete beneath her serape (Mike's *abuela*, I would find out later) stayed with me, guarding the kids. The men (Mike's father and uncle, I would find out later) stayed in the back of the truck, armed with the Remington and an arsenal of knives. We waited. The only sound I heard was the sound my own heart, knocking like a badly tuned engine.

And then they came limping in. No headlights, no taillights, no windshield – just a glittering rim of broken glass. Coughing and sputtering, the vehicle came to a stop about fifty yards from where I had parked the truck. The charred doors swung open and a burst of gunfire rang out, ricocheting off the rocks. The kids, the puppy, the grandma, all remained silent. I crouched outside the cave with my weapon drawn. Long minutes passed with no sound but the wind coming up, a mournful keening.

A whisper overhead, my heart jumped. I turned to look, pointing the pistol clutched between my hands. There on a ledge of rock above me, an owl, its heart-shaped face white in the star shine. We looked at each other, acknowledged each other. Both of us alive, hearts beating, sharing that particular slab of sandstone at that particular moment in time.

And then a new sound. In the distance a vibration like the hooves of a thousand buffalo thundering across the plains. Louder now, closer, the shaking of the earth became a throaty rumble, the sound of a dozen American-made motorcycles.

Tonto

Scattering swiftly, they surrounded the fort, leaving their steel ponies ground-tied and waiting. They were led by an old brave who had studied the ways of his ancestors and served in the occupier's recent wars. Tonto was no warrior, he was a medicine man.

His concern was for Kit and the children, but he also had Stormy to protect, not to mention the dude with the camera, the city slicker-reporter. Tonto didn't feel the lust for revenge in his soul, but he did own a desire to do good and the will to put things right. So many people to protect, it was a burden. But Tonto had a sharp knife, a well-strung bow, and a quiver of steel tipped, carbon fiber arrows. He might not have been quite as quick as he once was, but if anything, he was more experienced and far more sure.

A rapid burst of gunfire ripped through the rocks, it was hard to tell from where it came. His brothers and sisters would need time to evaluate the situation, to pinpoint their targets and get into position. The enemy had superior weaponry, but the Arapaho had strategy and stealth on their side.

"Let me be the bait," Stormy whispered in his ear, tugging his sleeve. "I can distract them for a minute, maybe draw them out of hiding."

Too risky. But she bolted, knowing her own mind, leaving the safety of his protection. Seeing a horizontal slab of rock nearby, she scrambled onto it. Shit. Nothing to do but cover her.

"Shine your light on me, honey," she called out. "Watch me groove."

Tonto swung the bike to face her, switching on the headlamp. Some of his tribe, hidden in the shadows, began a chant, their voices rising in unison. The sandstone amplified the sound until it became a true rock concert. Slowly she began to gyrate, peeling off her shirt one sleeve at a time, pulling her short leather skirt down over her hips and boots, stepping free of it, knowing she was being watched. Squatting, thrusting, spreading her limbs to their best advantage, she rhythmically contorted her near-naked body to the masculine chant as only Stormy Wether could do. Tonto himself was momentarily mesmerized. Meanwhile, under the cover of darkness, the other Arapahos crept in, raising their bows.

*

Kit

I heard the sound of Indian plainsong rising up from the ground itself. It was both earthy and bone-chilling eerie and the hair on my arms stood up. I kept my eyes alert for movement, ready to blow away anyone coming for my family. If this was to be the end of my world, I would go out in a firestorm, I would protect my kids with my last breath.

Gunfire nearby, instinctively I ducked bullets, and shards of rock went flying by my head. Then silence. The Indians had stopped chanting.

"Well looky here, if it ain't Kit Carson herself."

A man's voice with a Texas drawl. Definitely not Ratzer, who retained his nasal, East Coast twang. The Texan stepped out from behind a hoodoo, all boots, duster, and ten-gallon hat towering over me. I couldn't see his face.

"What do you want?" I spat.

"Hand over the whore. Give me that little bitch or you're all dead."

My blood rose up in rage and defiance. I was fixin' to shoot him, but I knew I only had one chance. My shot had to be true, it had to be right on the money. Aim for his heart, right in the center of his big, bloated chest. No time to raise the gun and line up the sight. Just point and squeeze all in one motion, hope to hell the slug finds its mark. That fat hombre would shoot me the instant I moved, I knew he would. It would be the last move I'd ever make.

I breathed one last time, a calmness coming over me. Then the man in the ten-gallon hat seemed to go all soft and tender. His knees buckled, and I watched in surprise as he withered, deflating like a giant lawn ornament, coming to rest on the ground in front of me, a feathered shaft in his side. In the rocks, the Indians started singing again – this time not a plainsong but a war cry.

*

When the dust settled, the sky was beginning to lighten. Three men lay face down in the dirt, hog-tied, beside the beaten black horse that had been their ride. The tires looked like pincushions, stuck with arrows, the feather fletching riffling in the wind.

Tonto and I were working to save their lives, the lives of the three men bleeding on the ground. We took care of a tension pneumothorax, a scalped head, and a broken femur, reduced and field-dressed them all nice and tidy. They would live to face trial.

Then, from the back seat, a tremendous fart – an explosion of wind passed in fear. Following the source, we found Bully Ratzer himself, cowering on the floorboard.

"Don't shoot me," he blathered.

We got him outside on the ground, in lithotomy position and hog-tied him with surgical tape for good measure.

"You're finished, Bully Boy," Balmy whispered in his ear as I pulled down his pants, exposing his quivering ass. "I'm exposing you to the world."

The reporter's camera clicked away. "Would you care to comment, Sheriff?"

"Unhand me, you bitches!"

"What most people don't realize is," I nurse-splained in a cheerful, condescending manner, "shit kills. And you, Sheriff Ratzer, are full of shit."

Balmy looked on as I snapped on a pair of gloves and chose the thickest rectal tube in the kit, inserted it into the brown-rimmed anus, inflating the balloon to keep it in place. Next I hooked up the enema bag, filled it with normal saline laced with chili pepper sauce and opened wide the infusion.

"That's what's called a triple-H enema, Balmy. Stands for High, Hot, and Helluvalot.

He cried like a baby, Bully Ratzer did.

On the eastern horizon the sun was a bleeding red gash.

*

The federal marshal had been notified, the Cheyenne medics were en route. The Electricans had taken a wheel off Ratzer's ride and siphoned his gas into my tank; we were ready to roll. I texted Doc Halliday an update. As per instructions, I had delivered the young dancer and saw her reunited with her sister under the protection of the Arapaho. I considered my mission accomplished.

"Good work, Carson," she answered. "The reward of a good deed done is the promise of another one to come. You're not done yet."

What sounded like an eagle's cry pierced the dawn, carrying over the rocks and plains. It was the tribal leader's signal; the warriors leaped to their wheeled ponies and took off, heading north on the highway in a thunderous roar.

Tonto helped me pack up the medical supplies. "Bring Balmy and follow us."

"Where? To the Wind River Reservation?"

He shook his head. "The Arapahos are nomads. We're going to see our cousins, the Sioux. There's a little matter about a pipeline they need our help with."

"Dakota territory? Look, I didn't even bring a change of clothes, I –"

"Hey, can I ride with you too?" Stormy said, getting off the back of Tonto's motorcycle. "That damn seat is killing my ass." The reporter asked to come along too, so he could get his story.

"I'm riding in the back with Mike and his family," said Wyatt. "Abuela's cooking up scrambled eggs, and I'm starving."

"Wait... They've got a kitchen back there?"

"Hot plates," Mike said. "Wired up to your battery."

"We better get charging, then."

The people in the back were no longer invisible, no longer nameless. They were the Trujillos: Angelina, Arturo, Ernesto, and Mike. We were a patchwork family, if only temporarily. We had each other's backs.

While the others jockeyed for their seats in the Power Wagon, Tonto and I embraced behind the sandstone hoodoo. It began as a warm hug of friendship and gratitude, but as I stepped away, he pulled me to him again and kissed me, long and deep, a kiss hot enough to set the prairie on fire.

"Stay with me, kemosabe," he said in my ear. "We'll figure this out."

I wanted to believe him. Somehow we'd find a way to make the West a good place to live again. Reluctantly we pulled apart, knowing this would continue. This would be consummated. I watched as he swung a leathered leg over the saddle, kick-started his mount and roared off, his long gray braid flying behind him. What the hell are you waiting for, Carson? I jumped in the cab, threw the Wagon in gear, peeling out in a shower of gravel and dust. Following my conscience, following my heart, following Tonto on the trail to Standing Rock. Drifting up from the back of the truck, the smell of fresh coffee and the sound of voices singing a new day's ballad.

***

More nurse fiction by L.S. Collison:

Friday Night Knife & Gun Club

Saturday Night Knife & Gun Club

Holiday on Planet Jolieterre: A Nova Skylar, Space Nurse Adventure

www.lindacollison.com

www.fictionhouseltd.com